HOMOEOPATHY FOR MIDWIVES

(and ALL PREGNANT WOMEN)

(2nd Edition)

BRITISH HOMOEOPATHIC ASSOCIATION
Patron: Her Majesty Queen Elizabeth The Queen Mother

WB 930
HOM   ALT MRD
MIDW

© 1999 British Homoeopathic Association

First published in 1992
Second Edition 1999
British Homoeopathic Association,
27A Devonshire Street,
London, W1N 1RJ

A Charity registered in England No. 235900

British Library Cataloguing in Publication Data.
A catalogue record for this book is available from the British Library.

ISBN No. 0 946717 702

ACKNOWLEDGEMENTS

Having completed this book I would like to express my gratitude to the following people who have all given me considerable help:

Enid Segall, General Secretary of the British Homoeopathic Association, encouraged me at the onset to start writing this book and has continued with helpful guidance and enthusiasm throughout.

Peggy and John Ainsworth, FRPharmS, who have helped greatly; Peggy with her typing skills on the 1st Edition and John on matters pharmaceutical and homoeopathic.

Janet Knowles, RGN, RM, read my final draft with the viewpoint of a midwife and made very helpful comments and suggestions.

Frances, whose patient understanding and diplomatic criticisms have been welcome and proved to be invaluable.

Finally, Mark, Victoria and Tristan who, with their good humour throughout, have helped in moments of difficulty.

CONTENTS

PREFACE TO 1st EDITION   vi

PREFACE TO 2nd EDITION   vii

Chapter 1 INTRODUCTION TO HOMOEOPATHY   1

What is homoeopathy

Remedies

Constitutional remedies

The use of the constitutional remedy in
midwifery practice

Selecting an 'ordinary' remedy

Chapter 2 THE PRE-CONCEPTION CLINIC   7

Chapter 3 FIRST ANTENATAL APPOINTMENT   8

Homoeopathic history taking

**Chapter 4 COMMON DIFFICULTIES IN THE FIRST
TRIMESTER**   10

Anaemia

Ectopic pregnancy

Fatigue

Heartburn

Miscarriages (threatened and inevitable)

Repeated miscarriages

Morning sickness

**Chapter 5 COMMON DIFFICULTIES IN THE SECOND
TRIMESTER**   17

Urogenital tract (vaginal discharge---recurrent thrush---
cystitis---incontinence of urine)

Abdominal symptoms (abdominal colic---constipation---
cravings---haemorrhoids)

Circulatory symptoms (cramps---fainting---palpitations---
phlebitis---varicose veins)

Skin changes

Miscellaneous (placenta praevia---abruptia placenta---
hydramnios---pre-eclampsia)

**Chapter 6 COMMON DIFFICULTIES IN THE THIRD
TRIMESTER, INCLUDING PREPARATION FOR
LABOUR with *Caulophyllum***   29

Backache

Braxton-Hicks' contractions

Emotional difficulties

Malpresentation

Preparation for labour with *Caulophyllum*

Chapter 7   **LABOUR**   **32**
              Hypotonic uterine activity
              Backache
              Analgesics
              After-pains
              Emergencies
Chapter 8   **SUMMARY - A SUGGESTED HOMOEOPATHIC**
              FRAMEWORK FOR PREGNANCY AND
              CHILDBIRTH   **35**
Chapter 9   **BREAST FEEDING DIFFICULTIES**   **36**
              Sore nipples
              Excessive breast milk production
              Loss of breast milk
              Mastitis
Chapter 10 **INFANT DIFFICULTIES IN THE NEONATAL**
              PERIOD   **39**
              Post labour
              Feeding difficulties
              Abdominal colic
              Septic spots
              Sticky eyes
              Night crying

BIBLIOGRAPHY   **43**

USEFUL INFORMATION AND ADDRESSES   **44**

INDEX   **48**

PREFACE (to 1st Edition)

This book is written to help midwives and all pregnant women understand how homoeopathy may be used to complement conventional midwifery skills and treatment, from the beginning of pregnancy through to the end of the postnatal period.

Homoeopathy is a totally safe method of therapeutics but it is important to remember it is not a magic medicine nor a panacea for all ills. If one is to use homoeopathy it must be based on a precise and informed diagnosis, as there are occasions when conventional therapy is the preferred approach.

Homoeopathy can be used in a purely complementary way with the skills and knowledge already used in pregnancy, childbirth and during the postnatal period.

Swan Acre
Sutton Courtenay

1992

PREFACE (to 2nd Edition)

This second Edition is written with some revised dosage schedules and additional homoeopathic remedies for conditions that were not included in the first Edition. This has been found necessary through wider clinical experience and through an attempted research project.

I have been actively pursuing a research project in the use of homoeopathic *Caulophyllum* in the antenatal period. The Professor of Obstetrics at the John Radcliffe Hospital agreed to head a triple blind trial using this remedy. The Senior Lecturer (Mr. William Ledger) worked out a protocol which was submitted to the government who had to give homoeopathic *Caulophyllum* a licence to be used as a 'drug'. This was successfully agreed. The ethical committee at the John Radcliffe Hospital agreed that the trial was satisfactory and all the consultant obstetricians agreed for the patients under their care to participate in the trial. The midwives at the John Radcliffe Hospital and in the community were enthusiastically wanting to participate in the trial, which was to be triple blind (active, placebo, and statistically blind).

Unfortunately, I was unable to obtain funding for this trial which therefore remains on the 'back burner'.

The Blackie Foundation Trust was involved in the preliminary discussions and, initially, were supportive of the trial but, when formally asked, gave a negative response. I then approached the MRC (Medical Research Council) who submitted the protocol to three (anonymous) referees. Two supported the trial and thought it timely but the third could not support the trial. The MRC operate on a unanimous verdict and not a majority.

I feel that this trial is important not only for homoeopathy but also for all pregnant women. *Caulophyllum* will shorten the length of labour, reduce the incidence of the use of an episiotomy, and will reduce the forceps delivery and caesarean section rates. If the trial were to show a statistically significant result, then it would help the cause of homoeopathy as well as the course of labour for all pregnant women.

There is anecdotal evidence that shows that this remedy is useful to use in preparation for labour. Dr. Janet Gray wrote to every medically qualified homoeopath in the U.K. for their experiences with *Caulophyllum*. Their experience was that it was useful with no adverse reactions. Animal work has also demonstrated its beneficial effect. Mr. Christopher Day, a homoeopathically-trained veterinary surgeon and the Veterinary Dean of the Faculty of Homoeopathy, has written a research project on pigs demonstrating its beneficial action. Anecdotal evidence of using *Caulophyllum* in cows, who have the same gestation period as for humans, shows a beneficial effect in the outcome of labour.

I hope that funding will be found so that this trial can be conducted.

I would like to thank Tristan for his consistent and patient help with computer matters in the writing of this 2nd Edition.

Finally, my grateful thanks go to Linda McCann for her dedication and editing skills.

Swan Acre
Sutton Courtenay

1999

CHAPTER 1

INTRODUCTION TO HOMOEOPATHY

1. What is Homoeopathy?

Homoeopathy was demonstrated as a method of therapeutics in 1806 by a German physician called Samuel Hahnemann. He found that by giving Peruvian Bark (Cinchona) to himself, he developed symptoms similar to those of people suffering from a local illness known as "marsh fever" (which is now known as malaria). He experimented on those people who were suffering from this fever by giving them this bark, which he had made into an alcoholic solution, and found that they recovered from the fever. This 'like cures like' fact led Hahnemann to use the term homoeopathy as a new method of therapy: from the Greek "homoeos" meaning similar and "pathos" meaning suffering.

2. Remedies

(a) How are remedies made?

The remedies are based on naturally occurring substances; common plants, insects, metals and their salts, seeds and snake venoms for example. They are crushed and prepared in alcoholic solution which is called the Mother Tincture. By diluting these solutions he was able to get rid of any previously noted side-effects.

In order to maintain a therapeutic action, his initial dilutions of one part in one hundred had to be vigorously shaken, a process called succussion.

Surprisingly, he noted that the weaker the solution became the stronger the homoeopathic/therapeutic effect became.

It is this basic homoeopathic principle that conventional doctors find difficult to accept.

This book uses the 6c and 30c potencies which are the centesimal dilutions (hence the letter 'c' after the remedy). One remedy prescribed in this book is in the dilution of the millesimal dilution which carries the letter 'M'. These very dilute solutions are made by diluting the original one in a hundred dilution a further one thousand times. They have the strongest homoeopathic/therapeutic effect. Continental Europe commonly uses the decimal dilution which is marked by the sign 'x'.

The remedies can be obtained in powder, granules, liquid (where the dose is two drops) or tablet form. There is no therapeutic difference between these: it is just a matter of personal preference.

The tablets and granules are lactose-based and so, if the pregnant woman has a lactose intolerance, she should ask for the preparations to be sucrose-based.

PREPARATION OF THE 6c POTENCY

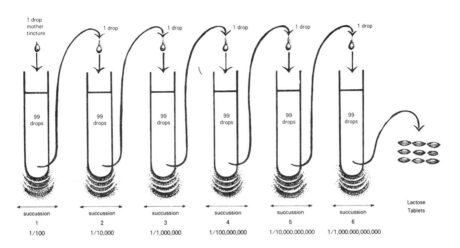

Remedies are written in Latin (this is a universal procedure) but, for the convenience of the midwife and the pregnant woman, the source of the remedy is given in brackets after the Latin name.

(b) How is the homoeopathic remedy taken?

Each remedy is sucked or chewed in the mouth and not swallowed. Ideally the remedy shouldn't be touched by hand (the hand may have substances on it that would inactivate the action of the remedy). Nothing should be eaten or drunk for at least 15 minutes before, or after, the remedy is placed within the mouth.

Remedies should be kept away from direct sunlight, heat and from strongly scented materials.

There are several substances that the woman should be advised not to take, whilst using the homoeopathic approach, as these will have a negative effect on the action of the remedy. These are caffeine (found in

2

chocolate, coffee and cola drinks), peppermint and codeine. Herbal teas are an appropriate drink, paracetamol or ibuprofen are suitable alternative non-codeine-containing analgesics and carob chocolate is a non-caffeine-containing chocolate.

(c) What is an aggravation?

Occasionally, the homoeopathic remedy may 'over-stimulate' the body causing a temporary deterioration of the symptoms. This is known as an aggravation. Although uncommon, it does show that the correct remedy has been selected and is not a cause for alarm. By immediately stopping the remedy, the aggravation will slowly subside and the woman will begin to feel better. If the aggravation is particularly severe, it can be stopped more quickly by drinking several cups of strong coffee. This will serve as an antidote to the remedy being used.

(d) What is a remedy picture?

Each remedy has certain specific effects on various parts and functions of the body. These have been noted by giving Mother Tinctures of each remedy to healthy volunteers and noting any symptoms that they may develop as a result. The profile of these symptoms for each remedy is known as its remedy picture.

The therapeutic application is to match the remedy picture that most closely matches the symptoms that a woman might be showing. Symptoms and the appropriate remedy can be found in a book called a Materia Medica.

This book gives common symptoms to be found at various stages of a pregnancy with their appropriate homoeopathic remedy.

3. Constitutional remedies

By recognizing our different likes and dislikes, both physical and emotional, it is possible to give these differences the qualities of 'symptoms'. This overall picture that is painted provides the so-called constitutional picture and the constitutional remedy.

The following are examples of constitutional pictures/remedies commonly to be found in midwifery practice.

ARGENTUM NITRICUM (silver nitrate)

This remedy picture describes a woman who has marked anticipatory anxiety. She is particularly fearful of heights and of crowds. She dislikes hot environments and desires sweet food to eat.

ARSENICUM ALBUM (arsenic trioxide)

This remedy picture describes an extremely neat and tidy woman who is also house-proud. She is very restless and is sensitive to the cold. Any symptoms that she may have are magnified out of all proportion. She enjoys sips of warm fluid. She feels worse at night, emotionally, and her physical symptoms tend to be worse at this late hour as well.

NATRUM MURIATICUM (sodium chloride)

This remedy picture describes a woman who has a greasy skin and characteristically has a crack in the middle of her lower lip. Outwardly, she gives the impression of being sociable but this conceals an inner shyness and a lack of confidence. She becomes easily distressed if she is left out of things. She is a woman who is able to bear a grudge against people who have offended her although, paradoxically, any attempt to console her will make her feel worse. Typically, she can be described as "nice to know but difficult to live with". She may suffer from throbbing migrainous headaches. She has a desire for salty foods and feels worse in both extremes of temperature (hot or cold).

NUX VOMICA (poison nut)

This remedy picture describes an ambitious woman, a high achiever who, because she is a perfectionist, finds difficulty, on becoming pregnant, in coping with the added stresses and strains of her life. She feels better in wet weather, provided that the rain is not associated with a cold wind. She has a desire for stimulants such as alcohol, coffee and, probably, cigarettes.

PHOSPHORUS

This remedy picture describes an emotionally sensitive woman who is able to give and to receive emotional support easily. She likes company and has an active social life. She probably has artistic qualities and may have a tint of red in her hair. She tends to tire easily, but responds quickly to short naps. She has a particular fear of thunderstorms.

PULSATILLA (wind-flower)

This remedy picture describes a woman who tends to cry easily and often. She particularly dislikes the heat which makes her feel very weak and prefers the fresh air, needing to keep her bedroom window open. She dislikes arguments, seeking harmony at all times. She is not particularly thirsty nor is she particularly emotionally demonstrative, much seeking to be supported emotionally and physically by someone else. She dislikes fatty foods and feels at her worse in the late afternoon.

SEPIA (inky juice of the cuttlefish)

This remedy picture describes a woman who feels completely overburdened by the situation and that no one else around her, particularly her husband, is pulling their weight to help her. She develops an indifference towards those people closest to her, preferring her own private space, away from all her loved ones. She feels tired all the time: sleep doesn't revive her but physical exercise, particularly dancing, does. Her tastes are for vinegary foods and "Marmite".

SULPHUR

This remedy picture describes a woman who has a ruddy complexion. She sweats easily and is forgetful; not particularly fussy about her personal appearance nor the tidiness of her surroundings. Her house has a lived-in feeling and she is always happy to have people around her. She enjoys a joke and has strong opinions about matters. She enjoys alcohol, particularly beer. She likes fatty foods but finds cow's milk disagrees with her.

4. The use of the constitutional remedy in midwifery practice

Firstly, it will boost the health of the woman staving off intercurrent illness, and help the symptom of **fatigue** commonly seen in the early stages of pregnancy.

Using the 30c potency, give one dose weekly reducing to a minimum of one a month, if the woman is able to tolerate this reduction: otherwise maintain the woman on the minimum dose that she finds will suit her.

Secondly, a 'constitutional' remedy can be used as an 'ordinary' remedy by using its 'organ specific' symptoms, found in its remedy picture, to treat certain illnesses during the antenatal period. The dosage schedules for these clinical illnesses will be shown in the appropriate chapter.

5.   Selecting an 'ordinary' remedy

In the following pages, remedies are named (with recommended dosage schedules) that may be helpful in clinical situations in midwifery practice.

If the remedy actually matches with the constitutional profile of the woman, then the therapeutic effect will be better.

Should there be no obvious match between the particular symptoms of the illness from the remedies described, then select the 'constitutional' remedy that most closely fits the woman as a whole, using the recommended dosage schedule for constitutional remedies.

CHAPTER 2

THE PRE-CONCEPTION CLINIC

Before conception, the woman should be made aware of the adverse effects of smoking on her planned pregnancy. It has been shown that smoking reduces placental blood flow to the baby and, therefore, it would not only be of benefit to the health of the mother-to-be but also to her baby. Referral to a counsellor may be helpful in order to support the woman in stopping smoking.

Her diet should also be discussed as it has been shown that a diet rich in folic acid (green-leafed vegetables and nuts), before conception, reduces neural tube abnormalities, notably spina bifida.

Conventional treatment is to advise the woman to take folic acid supplements before she decides to become pregnant. Once she is pregnant it will be too late to take folic acid supplements, as the beneficial effect of protecting against neural tube defects has been lost. Eating a diet rich in folic acid ensures an adequate intake of this important substance without taking a supplement.

It is also possible to take a homoeopathic remedy of folic acid as well, using the 6c potency. Take one dose, twice a day, as soon as the decision has been made to conceive.

She should also check, by means of a blood test, that she has antibody protection against German measles (rubella). If she has not, then active immunization is indicated before becoming pregnant.

CHAPTER 3

FIRST ANTENATAL APPOINTMENT

During this first important meeting, between the midwife and the pregnant woman, not only can the usual obstetric details be taken but it is also an opportunity to try and assess the woman homoeopathically.

Homoeopathic history taking

In the beginning, the homoeopathic approach will seem strange to the new homoeopathic midwife. The following breakdown of symptoms gives the indicated homoeopathic remedies.

(a) General symptoms

These assess the woman's reaction to certain environmental conditions and to her food likes and dislikes.

Feels worse in the heat	Argentum nitricum (silver nitrate)
	Natrum muriaticum (sodium chloride)
	Pulsatilla (wind-flower)
	Sulphur
Feels worse in the cold	Arsenicum album (arsenic trioxide)
	Nux vomica (poison nut)
Feels better in wet, warm weather	Nux vomica (poison nut)
Likes windy conditions	Sepia (inky juice of the cuttlefish)
Dislikes thunder	Phosphorus
Feels better in the fresh air	Pulsatilla (wind-flower)
	Phosphorus
Likes sweet foods and sweets	Argentum nitricum (silver nitrate)
	Sulphur
Dislikes fatty foods	Pulsatilla (wind-flower)
Likes fatty foods	Nux vomica (poison nut)
	Sulphur
Milk disagrees	Pulsatilla (wind-flower)
	Sulphur
	Sepia (inky juice of the cuttlefish)
Likes vinegar	Sepia (inky juice of the cuttlefish)
Likes salt	Argentum nitricum (silver nitrate)
	Natrum muriaticum (sodium chloride)

Feels worse in the early morning	Sulphur Nux vomica (poison nut)
Feels worse in the afternoon	Pulsatilla (wind-flower)
Feels worse late at night	Arsenicum album (arsenic trioxide)

(b) Mental symptoms

These describe the emotional side of the woman's personality.

Anxiety with a fear of heights and crowds	Argentum nitricum (silver nitrate)
Anxiety associated with marked restlessness	Arsenicum album (arsenic trioxide)
Short tempered, but quickly forgotten	Sulphur
Better for consolation	Pulsatilla (wind-flower)
Worse for consolation	Natrum muriaticum (sodium chloride)
Has a tendency to weep easily and often	Pulsatilla (wind-flower)
Ambitious, perfectionist	Nux vomica (poison nut)
Immaculately neat and tidy	Arsenicum album (arsenic trioxide)
Malleable, hates disharmony	Pulsatilla (wind-flower)

(c) Body appearance

As well as the symptoms classification, body appearance also provides pointers to a specific remedy.

Fair hair and blue eyes suggests	Pulsatilla (wind-flower)
Greasy hair and skin with a possible crack in the centre of the lower lip suggests	Natrum muriaticum(sodium chloride)
Ruddy complexion, sweaty and jolly, suggests	Sulphur
Sociable, and possibly artistic, with a hint of red in her hair suggests	Phosphorus

From all these clues an overall homoeopathic impression of the woman will be obtained, rather like painting a picture rather than taking a photograph. It doesn't matter if some of the clues don't absolutely fit.

This single remedy is known as the constitutional remedy. The way in which this can be used has been discussed in Chapter 1.

CHAPTER 4

COMMON DIFFICULTIES IN THE FIRST TRIMESTER

1. Anaemia

Excluding haemodilution, there are two types of anaemia seen in pregnancy, a microcytic anaemia that is due to iron deficiency (and a possible painless ectopic pregnancy) and a macrocytic anaemia due to a folate deficiency. These two anaemias must be determined by appropriate blood measurement assays and by careful examination, to exclude an ectopic pregnancy, in the case of an increasing microcytic anaemia in the presence of a normal blood iron measurement.

Provided that physical examination rules out the possibility of an ectopic pregnancy and because most women receive a sufficient iron and vitamin supply in their diet, giving every pregnant woman regular iron and vitamin supplements is considered unnecessary nowadays.

For some women, a regular supply of iron and folate supplements are considered necessary: notably if the woman has a past history of such an anaemia, or when the woman is carrying a multiple pregnancy or if, during the course of her pregnancy, she is found to have a genuine deficiency of iron or folate.

A homoeopathic approach can be helpful when a woman has a preference for this method of therapy and avoids the side-effects of the conventional medication (nausea and constipation).

The following homoeopathic remedies show pictures which are appropriate when they match with a particular woman. Using the 6c potency, give one dose twice a day.

Ferrum metallicum (iron)
This remedy picture describes a woman who is restless and has an aversion to eating eggs.

Ferrum phosphoricum (iron phosphate)
This remedy picture describes a woman who feels weak, who flushes easily and yet looks pale.

Folic acidum (folic acid)
This remedy picture has no specific symptoms and is only useful in those women who have been shown to have a folate deficiency.

2.   Ectopic pregnancy

This occurs when the fertilized egg becomes implanted in a place other than the uterus, usually one of the fallopian tubes. This causes considerable pain, then, as well as when the pregnancy breaks through the tube leading to a haemorrhage. Occasionally, the bleeding can go unrecognized and only presents as an increasing microcytic anaemia.

In both presentations this condition is life threatening, requiring immediate hospitalization for surgery.

The only homoeopathic remedy to be considered in this emergency situation is:

Aconitum napellus (monkshood)
> This remedy picture describes a sudden illness causing extreme anxiety with a fear of dying.
> Using the 30c potency, give one dose every 15 minutes while waiting for the ambulance.

Post operative management using homoeopathy

Arnica (leopard's bane)
> This remedy is useful for bruising that has occurred internally, as well as bruising extending externally from the operation.
> Using the 30c potency, give one dose immediately the woman has woken up from the anaesthetic. If there is a lot of bruising around the surgical wound, this remedy may be repeated in the same potency once more.

Hypericum (St. John's wort)
> This remedy can be given with *Arnica* as it will help the healing of the surgical scar. This remedy can be repeated in the same potency the following day.

Vitamin C (1000mgs) should be given daily, for one week, as this supplement will also help skin healing.

Staphysagria (stavesacre)
> This remedy should be given once, on the fourth post-operative day, using the 10M potency. It will help resolve any emotional disappointment that the woman may be feeling as a result of this disappointing outcome of her pregnancy. It will also physically help resolve any 'damage' to her urethra, should catheterization have taken place during the operation.

3. Fatigue

This common symptom and its homoeopathic treatment has already been discussed at the end of Chapter 1.

4. Heartburn

The following homoeopathic remedies may be helpful in treating heartburn, although many of the remedies used for treating early-morning sickness may also be helpful (provided that the remedy picture matches the symptoms that the woman is having).
Using the 6c potency, give one dose as required.

Homoeopathic remedies can also be used in conjunction with conventional antacids.

Asafoetida (gum of stinkasand)
> This remedy picture describes a woman who has marked flatulence and regurgitation. The woman may also have a tendency to behave irrationally.

Capsicum (cayenne pepper)
> This remedy picture particularly suits an obese woman who also notices a burning sensation on the tip of her tongue. She will be thirsty and, surprisingly, will find that drinking induces marked body shivering.

Carbo vegetabilis (vegetable charcoal)
> This remedy picture describes a woman who passes a great deal of wind both upwards and downwards. She feels worn-out and is improved when air is gently fanned over her face.

5. Miscarriage

This is defined as the loss of the foetus before the 18th week of pregnancy. At least 10-30% of all pregnancies end in miscarriage, usually before the 10th week. The symptoms are bleeding from the vagina, with or without cramping pains in the uterus. Miscarriages are classified as either threatened or inevitable. They are distinguished by vaginal examination.

If the os cervix is open, then the miscarriage is **inevitable**. In this situation, the contents of the uterus will be naturally rejected. If the bleeding is heavy, then hospital admission is indicated for a D and C.

Whilst waiting for the ambulance, the following homoeopathic remedy can be given:

Aconitum napellus (monkshood)
> This remedy picture describes extreme anxiety and fear.
> Using the 30c potency, give one dose immediately, and this dose may be repeated every fifteen minutes for a maximum of 6 doses.

If the os cervix is closed, then the miscarriage is **threatened** and the foetal heartbeat can be heard using an ultrasound.

Bed rest is advised, the heartbeat regularly listened for and, provided the heartbeat and the bleeding subsides, the woman can resume normal but gentle activity.

The following homoeopathic remedies may be used for a threatened miscarriage. Select one by matching its picture with the physical symptoms.

Aconitum napellus (monkshood)
> This remedy picture describes a woman who is showing extreme anxiety and has a particular fear of dying.
> Using the 30c potency, give one dose immediately and repeat every 15 minutes for a maximum of six doses.

Arnica (leopard's bane)
> This remedy should be used whenever there has been any injury preceding the miscarriage.
> Using the 30c potency, give one dose immediately and repeat twice at four hourly intervals.

Belladonna (deadly nightshade)
> This remedy picture describes a woman who has a red, flushed face. Her pulse rate is rapid and her pupils are dilated. Check that the woman is apyrexial (has no fever) and is not in shock, when immediate medical advice must be sought.
> Using the 30c potency, give one dose immediately and repeat three times at six hour intervals.

Ipecacuanha (ipecac-root)
> This remedy is indicated when the woman feels nauseated and may even vomit.
> Using the 30c potency, give one dose immediately and repeat, at hourly intervals, for a maximum of three doses.

Secale veratrum (ergot)
>This remedy picture describes blood loss that is profuse and blackish, leaving the woman feeling weak, exhausted, and fearful of dying. Clearly, the woman in this clinical state must be assessed by a medical practitioner.
>
>When using this remedy, it is important to regularly check the os because, although the bleeding subsides, the cervix might have opened, in which case the miscarriage has become inevitable. In this case, follow the advice for an inevitable miscarriage.
>
>If the os remains closed, then the remedy may be used in the 30c potency giving one dose immediately and repeating, with caution, daily, for a maximum of three doses.

6. Repeated miscarriages

This situation needs a detailed gynaecological investigation to check that there are no genetic, hormonal or uterine abnormalities. Provided that there are no abnormalities, then the following homoeopathic remedies can be used.

Select one of them by matching its picture with the clinical symptoms and, using the 6c potency, give one dose twice a day.

Caulophyllum (blue cohosh)
>This remedy picture describes a woman who has recurrent miscarriages. She may feel needle-like pains in her cervix. She may also experience severe drawing-like pains in the small joints of her fingers and toes.

Sepia (inky juice of cuttlefish)
>This remedy picture has a special affinity for the uterus and helps the foetus stay within it. The remedy is primarily selected from the general picture of the woman. She is a woman who prefers her own space, and easily goes off those closest to her. She likes vinegar, 'Marmite' and fresh, sunny, windy weather. She prefers warmth as she is sensitive to the cold.

7. Morning sickness

Nausea and vomiting is common in early pregnancy, usually starting before the sixth week and discontinuing at about the twelfth week, although it may continue throughout the pregnancy. It generally occurs early in the morning, on waking, although it can happen at any time of the day.

Sufferers may find that it is relieved if they are able to eat little and often rather than the normal breakfast, lunch and evening meal.

Conventional treatment has little to offer in the form of safe drug therapy.

The following homoeopathic remedies can be used quite safely to help reduce this symptom. Select one of them by matching its picture with the physical symptoms. Using the 6c potency, give one dose three times a day.

Arsenicum album (arsenic trioxide)

This remedy picture describes a woman whose sickness is also probably associated with diarrhoea. Generally the woman is chilly, thirsty, anxious and exceptionally neat and tidy: she is house proud.

Ipecacuanha (ipecac-root)

This remedy picture describes a woman who feels nauseated all the time: even vomiting doesn't bring any relief from this symptom.

Natrum muriaticum (sodium chloride)

This remedy picture describes a woman with morning sickness who also has a craving for salt. She has greasy skin and a characteristic crack in the centre of her lower lip. She is generally shy, but overcomes this by creating an artificial sense of gaiety. She is very sensitive to loud noises and easily bears a grudge against anyone who crosses her path. Typically, she can be described as a woman who is "nice to know, but difficult to live with".

Nux vomica (poison nut)

This remedy picture describes a woman with morning sickness, whose abdomen feels bloated and is particularly tender to firm pressure. When she belches, she gets a bitter taste in her mouth. The woman is ambitious, a perfectionist and enjoys alcohol and coffee. She possibly finds it difficult to stop smoking or eating chocolates (which contain caffeine).

Phosphorus

This remedy picture describes a woman whose nausea and vomiting are worse towards evening. It may be brought on by eating salty foods and by eating cold foods and fluids, which are vomited as they warm up in her stomach. This remedy describes a woman who is fearful of thunder, has a wide circle of friends, tires easily but quickly revives after a short nap.

Pulsatilla (wind-flower)

This remedy picture describes a woman who becomes nauseated when eating or smelling fatty foods. She feels better in the fresh air and worse in hot environments. She weeps easily and responds well to a reassuring cuddle. She can cause concern because she doesn't want to take fluids readily.

Sepia (inky juice of the cuttlefish)

This is the classic remedy for morning sickness as the remedy picture describes a woman who feels sick at the sight, smell or even the thought of food. However, this symptom is improved when she eats or drinks in small amounts. She is a woman who feels most comfortable in her own space, and can become depressed if this space is denied her.

CHAPTER 5

COMMON DIFFICULTIES IN THE SECOND TRIMESTER

1. Urogenital tract

(a) Vaginal discharge

It is important to make an accurate diagnosis of any vaginal discharge by taking swabs and urine cultures, so that a conventional treatment can be used. The following homoeopathic remedies can be given whilst awaiting the laboratory reports, or when these reports give negative results and yet the symptoms remain.

Matching the clinical symptoms with the correct remedy picture, give the 6c potency, four times a day for four days, reducing to twice a day if the reports are negative and the remedy is to be used as a long term form of treatment.

Hydrastis (golden seal)
> This remedy picture describes a thick, ropey discharge that causes marked pruritis vulvae.

Kreosotum (beechwood kreosote)
> This remedy picture describes a discharge that is particularly smelly and stains her underwear a dark colour.

Nitricum acidum (nitric acid)
> This remedy picture describes a vaginal discharge that causes a pricking sensation in her vagina which may also be ulcerated.

Pulsatilla (wind-flower)
> This remedy picture describes a vaginal discharge that is bland in colour and non-irritant.

Sepia (inky juice of the cuttlefish)
> This remedy picture describes a vaginal discharge that is jelly-like. The woman may feel that her vagina is prolapsed and for this reason prefers to sit with her legs crossed. She can become moody, retiring into her own space. Things can get on top of her, and she can emotionally switch off those people closest to her.

(b) Recurrent thrush

This can be a frequently recurring infection with the yeast-like fungus called candida albicans. When this occurs the woman (and her sexual partner), having had adequate conventional treatment, should be encouraged to reduce her intake of refined sugar as this creates a favourable environment in which candida albicans thrives.

If conventional treatment fails, then the following homoeopathic remedies can be considered (as well as those remedies listed above for vaginal discharge). Select the remedy by matching its picture with the clinical symptoms.

Helonias (unicorn root)

This remedy picture describes a woman who has a copious vaginal discharge causing marked irritation and itchiness of the whole of her vulva, which becomes swollen and tender. The woman herself becomes miserable and can only cope by keeping herself busy. Using the 6c potency, give one dose, twice a day, for up to two weeks.

Candida albicans

If the vaginal swab shows that the discharge is due to candida albicans, that hasn't responded to conventional treatment, and none of the above remedy pictures fits, then it is possible to take a homoeopathic remedy derived from *Candida albicans*. Using the 6c potency, give one dose, twice a day, for two weeks.

(c) Cystitis

It is important to make an accurate diagnosis by checking midstream samples of urine and to treat any bacterial infection conventionally. The following remedies may be used to help treat the irritating symptoms whilst waiting for the laboratory results. In many cases, the homoeopathic treatment will have cured the infection.

Drinking barley water frequently will also help to soothe the initial dysuria (pain occurring towards the end of urination). If the woman suffers from recurrent urine infections, then drinking regular cranberry juice will help to keep the urine sterile.

Select the homoeopathic remedy by matching its picture with the clinical symptoms. Using the 6c potency, give one dose, twice a day, for up to five days.

Cantharis (spanish fly)

This remedy picture describes violent irritation in the bladder causing frequency, urgency and dysuria.

Sarsaparilla (smilax)

This remedy picture describes terminal dysuria.

Staphysagria (stavesacre)

This remedy picture describes pain along the urethra which is eased when the woman passes urine. This remedy is indicated for urine infections caused through sexual intercourse and after catheterisation.

(d) Incontinence of urine

A pregnant woman can become incontinent of urine whenever she coughs, sneezes or lifts anything heavy. This annoying symptom can be helped by one of the following homoeopathic remedies.

Select one by matching its picture with the physical symptoms. Using the 6c potency, give one dose, twice a day, for one week, reducing the frequency to once a day.

Causticum (Hahnemann's mixture of quicklime (calcium oxide) with potassium bisulphate)

This remedy picture describes a woman who finds it difficult to start passing urine, and may go into a state of "retention of urine". She more commonly suffers from stress incontinence.

Natrum muriaticum (sodium chloride)

This remedy picture describes a woman who suffers from stress incontinence of urine but also finds it difficult to micturate in the presence of other people.

The general profile of the woman homoeopathically, as described in Chapter 1, will help in the selection of this remedy.

Pulsatilla (wind-flower)

This remedy picture describes a woman who suffers from stress incontinence whenever she laughs, cries or passes flatus.

The general profile of the woman homoeopathically, as described in Chapter 1, will help in the selection of this remedy.

2. Abdominal symptoms

(a) Abdominal colic

This symptom of intermittent abdominal pain must be accurately diagnosed so that an acute abdomen is not missed. The pains can arise from constipation or diarrhoea. Having satisfied oneself that there is no acute abdomen, the following homoeopathic remedies can be safely given. Match the remedy picture with the clinical symptoms. Using the 6c potency, give one dose, twice a day, for a maximum of one week.

Colocynthis (bitter cucumber)

This remedy picture describes colicky pain that forces the woman to bend over double. It is this firm pressure that relieves the pain. Generally the woman tends to be irritable and angry.

Magnesium phosphoricum (magnesium phosphate)

This remedy picture describes colicky abdominal pain that is relieved much more by warmth than by firm pressure.

(b) Constipation

It is important for a pregnant woman, who becomes constipated, to resolve this difficulty using dietary means rather than resort to proprietary laxatives. The diet should include as much fibre as possible as well as an adequate amount of fluid. There are a number of 'natural' laxatives:

'Syrup of figs',

dried fruits (particularly apricots and prunes),

linseed soaked in boiled water and drunk as a herbal tea, two or three times a day (linseed can also be sprinkled on breakfast cereals or into soups), and

molasses (black treacle) 10-15ml (2-3 teaspoons) to be taken, three times a day, as it comes or spread on food.

Probiotic supplements can also be safely taken, as these help restore the micro-flora of the gastrointestinal tract and, therefore, help restore normal bowel activity.

The following homoeopathic remedies can also be used in conjunction with the above advice. Match the remedy picture with the clinical symptoms and, using the 6c potency, give one dose daily.

Alumina metallicum (aluminium)

This remedy picture describes a pregnant woman who has lost all expulsive power to defecate despite having the urge to do so. An unusual symptom that she may have (and this is very significant from a homoeopathic point of view) is that potatoes disagree with her.

Nux vomica (poison nut)

This remedy picture describes a pregnant woman who has a frequent desire to defecate but is always left feeling as though her rectum has never been properly emptied.

The general profile of the woman, as described in Chapter 1, may help in the selection of this remedy.

Silicea (pure flint)

This remedy picture describes a stool that appears, only to retreat back into the anus - the so-called "bashful stool".

The general profile of the woman that this remedy suits, is that she appears to lack confidence and has a general lack of 'go', is forgetful, just letting life drift by. However, when particularly irritated, she can lose her temper. She also sweats easily from her feet.

(c) Cravings

Some women, at this stage of pregnancy, can develop a craving for certain types of food. Whilst this is not a problem in itself (some find it a joke), the woman and her family may consider it to be a problem.

The following homoeopathic remedies are applicable to a woman who has a particular craving for a specific food. Using the 30c potency, give one dose every time that the woman experiences the craving.

Beer and brandy	Nux vomica (poison nut)
Caffeine	Angostura vera (bark of Galipea Cusparia)
Chocolate	Nux vomica (poison nut)
Cigarettes	Nux vomica (poison nut)
Eggs	Calcarea carbonica (calcium carbonate)
Fat	Acid nitricum (nitric acid)
Ice cream	Phosphorus
Oysters	Lachesis (bushmaster snake venom)
Raw food	Sulphur
Refined sugar	Sulphur
Salt	Natrum muriaticum (sodium chloride) or Phosphorus. The general profile of the woman from a homoeopathic point of view, as described

	in Chapter 1, will help to distinguish between these two remedies.
Smoked food	Causticum (Hahnemann's mixture of quicklime (calcium oxide) with potassium bisulphate)
'Strange' food	Lyssin (saliva from a rabid dog). The woman may also do strange things in her behaviour.
Sweet food	Argentum nitricum (silver nitrate) or China (Peruvian bark) or Lycopodium (club moss). The remedy picture for *Argentum nitricum* is a person who dislikes warm, crowded atmospheres and has a fear of heights. The remedy picture for *China* is of a person who feels exhausted from loss of body fluids, possibly sweats, or a woman who is recovering from an intercurrent illness. The *Lycopodium* picture describes a woman who has an anticipatory anxiety that, in reality, is baseless. She feels at her worse between 4pm and 8pm.
Vinegar	Sepia (inky juice of the cuttlefish)
Whisky	Sulphur
Wine	Phosphorus or Sulphur. The general homoeopathic profiles, described in Chapter 1, will help distinguish between these two remedies.

(d) Haemorrhoids

This condition is common in all pregnant women as their babies grow in their abdomen, causing pressure to build up in the veins around their anuses. This can cause bleeding and/or irritation. It is important to check that the woman is not constipated and, therefore, straining to defecate.

The following homoeopathic remedies can be given to treat the haemorrhoids directly. Select the remedy picture that most closely matches the symptoms of the woman and, using the 6c potency, give one dose three times a day for a maximum of two weeks, reducing the dose to a minimum to keep the symptoms under control.

Aesculus hippocastanum (horse chestnut)
This remedy picture describes haemorrhoids that give sharp shooting pains that radiate up the woman's back.

Nux vomica (poison nut)

This remedy picture describes a woman who feels that her rectum is never properly emptied whenever she defecates. Her haemorrhoids may or may not bleed.

The general profile of this woman is helpful when selecting this remedy. This is described in Chapter 1.

Paeonia (peony)

This remedy is used as an ointment, to be used as often as required. The remedy picture describes very itchy haemorrhoids, causing a burning feeling particularly after the woman has defecated.

Sulphur

This remedy picture describes haemorrhoids that bleed producing a burning and itchy feeling in her anus. The woman also has painless diarrhoea in the morning, which often forces her to rush out of bed to the toilet.

The general homoeopathic profile of the woman, as described in Chapter 1, will help in the selection of this remedy.

3.   Circulatory problems

(a) Cramps

Cramps in the lower limbs can cause much distress. They can be associated with varicose veins, in which case the woman should be advised to wear support stockings. For other causes, the following homoeopathic remedies can be used.

Using the 6c potency, give one dose immediately. If the cramps occur regularly, give one dose, twice a day, as a preventive measure.

Select the appropriate remedy by matching the clinical features with the remedy picture.

Arnica (leopard's bane)

This remedy picture describes a pregnant woman whose legs develop cramps and the legs always feel tired.

Coffea cruda (unroasted coffee)

This remedy picture describes a woman who easily develops cramps. She is over-active and finds it difficult to get to sleep, tossing around, unable to relax.

Cuprum metallicum (copper)
>This remedy picture describes a woman who develops cramps that come in repeated spasms. This remedy can be combined with *Chamomilla* (camomile) which can be given at monthly intervals by injection (deep subcutaneous). This preparation is useful when *Cuprum metallicum,* whilst indicated, is not working on its own.

Nux vomica (poison nut)
>This remedy is for a pregnant woman who develops cramps in her calf muscles and also in the soles of her feet. Her arms have a tendency to 'go to sleep'.
>The general profile of the woman, as described in Chapter 1, will help in the selection of this remedy.

(b) Fainting
It is important to correctly establish that the diagnosis is a simple faint and not an epileptic fit.

Provided that it is a simple faint, the following homoeopathic remedies can be used to help prevent it from recurring. Select the remedy by matching its picture with the clinical symptoms and, using the 6c potency, give one dose following the faint and repeat the dose, daily, for the following week.

Aconitum napellus (monkshood)
>This remedy picture describes a woman who has fainted, and wakes up feeling anxious and fearful of dying.

Belladonna (deadly nightshade)
>This remedy picture describes a woman who faints whenever she gets hot, either from a warm atmosphere or from a fever.

Carbo vegetabilis (vegetable charcoal)
>This remedy picture describes an obese woman who sweats easily and generally feels worn-out. She faints easily and often responds well by having cool air fanned over her face.

China (Peruvian bark)
>This remedy picture describes a woman who sweats easily and heavily and, as a result of losing body fluid, becomes exhausted and faints. She is sensitive to the slightest touch, from any draught, and is improved by warmth and the open air.

Ignatia (St.Ignatius' bean)
> This remedy picture describes a woman who faints easily from any form of unhappiness, especially grief.

(c) Palpitations
> This form of heart irregularity must be accurately diagnosed, as conventional treatment might be the more appropriate treatment.
> If the palpitations are causing the woman emotional problems, but have been accurately diagnosed as being not medically serious, then homoeopathic treatment can be safely used. Select the one that most closely fits the symptoms. Using the 6c potency, give one dose twice a day.

Aconitum napellus (monkshood)
> This remedy picture describes a woman who develops palpitations from an emotional shock or because of great anxiety.

Arsenicum album (arsenic trioxide)
> This remedy picture describes a woman who tends to develop palpitations towards midnight and whenever she lies on her right side. Their recurrence is reduced by her keeping calm.
> The general profile of the woman, as described in Chapter 1, will help in the selection of this remedy.

Lycopodium (club moss)
> This remedy picture describes a woman whose palpitations begin between 4pm-8pm and when she lies on her left side.
> The profile of the woman that this remedy will suit has an anticipatory anxiety, is fearful of being left on her own and feels better from being uncovered, in order to cool down.

Pulsatilla (wind-flower)
> This remedy picture describes a woman who develops palpitations after eating rich, fatty foods and, also, when in hot environments.
> The general features of the remedy, as described in Chapter 1, will help in the selection of this remedy.

(d) Phlebitis
> Treatment with support stockings is indicated, in association with the following homoeopathic remedies for varicose veins. Select the remedy by matching its picture with the clinical symptoms.

Using the 6c potency, give one dose three times a day, initially for two weeks, reducing to one 6c dose, twice a day.

(e) Varicose veins

These appear in some women as a result of the extra pressure in their abdomen, which causes the veins of their legs to become more prominent. The initial treatment is with support stockings. The following homoeopathic remedies will also help in reducing their size. Using the 6c potency, give one dose twice a day.

Arsenicum album (arsenic trioxide)

This remedy picture describes a woman who develops varicose veins.

The general homoeopathic profile of the woman, as described in Chapter 1, will help in the selection of this remedy.

Carbo vegetabilis (vegetable charcoal)

This remedy picture describes a woman whose varicose veins have a tendency to ulcerate.

The woman feels faint, probably from the loss of body fluid (sweat). She feels worse when her face is gently fanned with cold air.

Fluoricum acidum (hydrofluoric acid)

This remedy picture describes a woman who develops varicose veins and has a sensation as if hot water was coming out of all the sweat pores of her leg.

Hamamelis virginica (witch-hazel)

This remedy picture describes a woman who has developed varicose veins and whose leg muscles feel tired. She also has a cold sensation running down the backs of her legs and neuralgic pains going down the inside of both legs.

Pulsatilla (wind-flower)

This remedy picture describes a woman who develops painful varicose veins. She produces a cold sweat on her legs, and her feet produce a foul-smelling sweat. Her legs become numb whenever she stands for long periods.

The general homoeopathic profile of the woman, as described in Chapter 1, will help in the selection of this remedy.

Sepia (inky juice of the cuttlefish)

> This remedy picture describes a woman with varicose veins who has the sensation that a mouse is running up and down her legs. The general homoeopathic profile of the remedy picture, as described in Chapter 1, will help in the selection of this remedy.

4. Skin changes

When a woman becomes pregnant, she may notice certain skin changes, particularly on her face, and this is called chloasma. It is due to an increase of circulating oestrogens. They rarely cause any problems but the following homoeopathic remedies can be used if they become troublesome. Using the 6c potency, give one dose daily.

Arsenicum album (arsenic trioxide)

> This remedy picture describes a woman whose scalp becomes so sensitive that she finds it difficult to comb or brush her hair. The general homoeopathic profile of the woman, as described in Chapter 1, will help in the selection of this remedy.

Lachesis (bushmaster snake venom)

> This remedy picture describes a woman whose skin develops purple blotches on it, which become more prominent when she wakes up in the morning.

Nux vomica (poisoned nut)

> This remedy picture describes a woman whose skin problems are worsened whenever she drinks coffee or alcohol. The general homoeopathic profile of the woman, as described in Chapter 1, will help in the selection of this remedy.

Sepia (inky juice of the cuttlefish)

> This remedy picture describes a freckly rash, shaped like a butterfly, which appears over her nose and spreads across to her cheeks. The general homoeopathic profile of the woman, as described in Chapter 1, will help in the selection of this remedy.

Sulphur

> This remedy picture describes a woman who has a dry skin that worsens whenever she washes her face. She tends to blush easily.

The general homoeopathic profile of the woman, as described in Chapter 1, will help in the selection of this remedy.

5. Miscellaneous

Placenta praevia, abruptia placenta, hydramnios, and pre-eclampsia. All of these conditions are best treated conventionally.

However, homoeopathy can be used in conjunction with conventional treatment.

To allay any anxiety (see emotional problems), use her constitutional remedy if applicable to the mother (see Chapter 1 for possible constitutional pictures).

If delivery is by caesarean section, then the homoeopathic remedies of *Arnica* (leopard's bane), *Hypericum* (St. John's wort) and *Staphysagria* (stavesacre) can be used, in the potencies described in the section on ectopic pregnancy.

CHAPTER 6

COMMON DIFFICULTIES IN THE THIRD TRIMESTER INCLUDING THE PREPARATION FOR LABOUR
with Caulophyllum

1. Backache

Some women find this a problem at this stage of their pregnancy. The following homoeopathic remedies can be used to help. Select one by matching the remedy picture with the clinical symptoms.

Using the 30c potency, one dose should be sufficient to ease the backache. If it isn't, then use the 6c potency and give one dose, twice a day, for up to one week.

Bellis perennis (daisy)

This remedy picture describes a woman who suffers from generalized muscle aches, particularly in her back and the front of her thighs, which makes walking difficult.

Kali carbonicum (potassium carbonate)

This remedy picture describes a woman who develops pain in the small of her back, which radiates into both of her hips. The symptoms change with the weather, being worse in the cold; particularly cold winds.

Natrum muriaticum (sodium chloride)

This remedy picture describes a woman whose pain in the small of her back is relieved by firm pressure.

The general homoeopathic profile of this remedy, as discussed in Chapter 1, will help in the selection of this remedy.

Rhus toxicodendron (poison ivy)

This remedy picture describes a woman whose backache is worse whenever she begins to move, improving on subsequent movement. The pain returns when she becomes tired. She tends to be a restless woman, because she is aware that movement does help the backache. She also knows that the pain is relieved by warmth.

2. Braxton-Hicks' contractions

These pains are not labour contractions but they can cause the woman distress. The following homoeopathic remedy will help reduce the frequency of these pains.
Using the 6c potency, give one dose daily.

Cimicifuga racemosa (black snake root)
This remedy picture describes shooting pains that radiate across the woman's abdomen.

3. Emotional difficulties

Any emotional difficulty is best managed by good listening and midwifery skills, but the following homoeopathic remedies can be safely used as a method of support therapy.
Select the remedy whose picture most closely matches the clinical symptoms. Using the 30c potency, give one dose daily for one week reducing the dose to one, weekly.

Aconitum napellus (monkshood)
This remedy picture describes a woman who has a major unresolved anxiety that continues to escalate as the expected delivery date gets closer. She is fearful of dying.

Argentum nitricum (silver nitrate)
This remedy picture describes a woman who, even before she became pregnant, had a generalized anxiety that causes her to have frequency of micturition. She has a desire for sweets, a fear of heights and crowded places, and a general dislike of hot environments.

Arnica (leopard's bane)
This remedy picture describes a woman who becomes fearful of pain at her forthcoming labour. Generally, she is a woman who is probably agoraphobic preferring to be left on her own.

Arsenicum album (arsenic trioxide)
This remedy picture describes a woman who is exceptionally neat and tidy and who has marked anxiety associated with restlessness. She is sensitive to the cold, feeling cold all the time and is thirsty, but only for sips of fluid at a time. There is a deterioration of all

these symptoms towards midnight.

Gelsemium (yellow jasmine)
This remedy picture describes a woman who has a marked anticipatory anxiety that give her 'butterflies in her stomach': it is as if she is going to take an examination every day. She prefers to be left on her own, and may cause the midwife concern because of her lack of thirst.

4.   Malpresentation

If, at this stage of pregnancy, the presentation is not vertex and the obstetrician has deemed it necessary to correct the presentation, by external version, the following homoeopathic remedy will help maintain the foetus in its corrected position.

Pulsatilla (wind-flower)
This remedy should be given in the 6c potency, twice a day.

If the presentation is unstable, or even a breech, then the same remedy, using the same potency and dosage, will encourage the foetus to adopt the correct position, preventing the need for medical intervention.

5.   Preparation for labour with *Caulophyllum*.

At the 37th week, a pregnant woman should start taking the following homoeopathic remedy. It makes for an easier labour by strengthening uterine muscular activity and softening the os cervix. This means that the foetus descends more quickly, reducing the incidence of an episiotomy, or a forceps or caesarean section delivery.
Using the 30c potency, give one dose twice a week (but not on consecutive days) until labour starts.

Caulophyllum (blue cohosh)
This remedy picture describes extreme rigidity of the os cervix and weak uterine muscular activity during labour.
The remedy can also be given as a single 30c potency dose, if labour pains begin to diminish.
The remedy picture also describes stiffness of the small joints of the fingers and toes.
This remedy classically describes the homoeopathic principle of 'like cures like'.

CHAPTER 7

LABOUR

Every woman should already have the following homoeopathic remedies easily to hand, to be used initially and when in hospital or during a home delivery. The remedies should all be in the 30c potency except for Staphysagria (stavesacre) which is in the 10M potency.

Arnica (leopard's bane) and *Hypericum* (St. John's wort) should be taken as soon as established labour has taken place.

The *Arnica* will reduce blood loss and bruising. It will also stop a precipitate labour. The *Hypericum* will help heal any vulval damage and, in the unlikely event of an episiotomy, it will help skin healing. In the even more unlikely event of a forceps delivery, it will help reduce any sacral pain and, if a caesarean section is needed, it will help skin healing.

Staphysagria (stavesacre) should be taken on the 4th post partum day. It will help the woman adjust to any disappointments she may be feeling if her birth plan didn't follow her wishes and prevent 'post partum blues'. It will also help 'heal' the urethra should catheterization have taken place during delivery.

1. Hypotonic uterine activity

If the uterine contractions diminish in a woman, who was previously in established labour, the following homoeopathic remedies can be given as separate doses (30c potency) to help re-establish labour.

The first choice is Caulophyllum (blue cohosh).
The second choice is Natrum muriaticum (sodium chloride).
The third choice is Pulsatilla (wind-flower).

2. Backache

Natrum muriaticum (sodium chloride)
> given as a single 30c dose. This is particularly helpful with a posterior presentation.

3. Analgesics in labour

These homoeopathic remedies can be used with 'gas and air'. Using the 30c potency, give a single dose.

Belladonna (deadly nightshade)

> This remedy picture describes a woman who is red-faced, moaning, and whose thoughts and behaviour may have become irrational. The labour pains come and go frequently.

Chamomilla (German chamomile)

> This remedy picture describes a woman who says "I can't bear the pain". As well as giving this remedy, the woman responds to being cuddled and made to feel as if she is being carried.

Cimicifuga racemosa (black snake-root)

> This remedy picture describes a woman who says "I can' t do it" and wants to give up. She becomes increasingly agitated, and may develop visions of rats and mice.

4. After-pains

These gripeing pains in the uterus can follow delivery. The following homoeopathic remedies can be given as a single 30c potency dose. Select the correct remedy by matching its picture with the clinical symptoms.

Caulophyllum (blue cohosh)

> This is the first choice of the remedies and is particularly useful where the labour has been prolonged.

Sabina (savine)

> This remedy picture describes intense after-pains that feel worse for the least movement and better when the windows of her room are wide open, allowing cool, fresh air to enter.

Secale (ergot)

> This remedy picture describes a woman with after-pains that are worse when she is covered with the bedclothes and are relieved when she is lying on her back, exposed.

5. Emergencies

In these two extremely serious conditions, homoeopathic remedies should only be given after calling an obstetrician for urgent help:

(a) Retained placenta
Sabina (savine)
>This remedy can be given, as a single 30c potency, to help the normal expulsion of the placenta, following delivery. If successful, it would make a manual extraction unnecessary.

(b) Post partum haemorrhage
When the amount of blood loss, following delivery, exceeds 200mls or when vaginal bleeding continues, following delivery of the placenta, the woman is said to be suffering post partum haemorrhage.

The following homoeopathic remedies can only be given after the obstetrician has been called.

Phosphorus
>This remedy should be given as a single 30c potency dose. Its remedy picture describes profuse uterine haemorrhage. The overall homoeopathic picture of the woman, as described in Chapter 1, will decide in the selection of this remedy.

Secale (ergot)
>This remedy should be given as a single 30c potency dose. Its remedy picture describes stopping uterine blood loss. The woman feels unhappy by being covered with bed-clothes, because of their warmth, and so she pushes them away, preferring to lie exposed, particularly on her back.

CHAPTER 8

SUMMARY

A SUGGESTED HOMOEOPATHIC FRAMEWORK FOR PREGNANCY AND CHILDBIRTH

1. **The first antenatal appointment**

    Explanation of the homoeopathic principles, and the method of taking remedies.
    Explanation of substances that can diminish the homoeopathic effect.
    An appraisal of the woman's homoeopathic symptoms leading to the evaluation of the appropriate constitutional remedy.

2. **Explanation of the treatment of difficulties that may develop during the antenatal period, and the use of *Caulophyllum* from the 37th week.**

3.   **Labour**

    Essential remedies to be taken at the onset of labour
    > Arnica (leopard's bane) 30c
    > Hypericum (St. John's wort) 30c

    Other remedies to have close at hand
    > Belladonna (deadly nightshade) 30c
    > Caulophyllum (blue cohosh) 30c
    > Chamomilla (German chamomile) 30c
    > Cimicifuga racemosa (black snake root) 30c
    > Hypericum (St. John's wort) 30c
    > Natrum muriaticum (sodium chloride) 30c
    > Phosphorus 30c
    > Pulsatilla (wind-flower) 30c
    > Sabina (savine) 30c
    > Secale (ergot) 30c
    > Staphysagria (stavesacre) 10M

CHAPTER 9

BREAST FEEDING DIFFICULTIES

1. Sore nipples

The homoeopathic and conventional treatment is to use nipple shields and to apply creams to soften the nipples. The homoeopathic cream is calendula (marigold) applied as often as necessary.

The following homoeopathic remedies can also be taken orally. Using the 30c potency, give one dose immediately, followed by the 6c potency daily, until the problem is resolving. Select the remedy by matching its picture with the clinical symptoms.

Chamomilla (German chamomile)
> This remedy picture describes nipples that are inflamed, making the nipples so tender that the woman prevents her baby from sucking from them. In this situation, the mother becomes increasingly irritable.

Nitric acidum (nitric acid)
> This remedy picture describes nipples that are very cracked so that, when her baby suckles from them, the mother feels a severe pricking sensation as if splinters were piercing her nipples.

2. Excessive breast milk production

The following homoeopathic remedies can be given to those mothers who are producing too much milk. Select the remedy by matching its picture with the clinical symptoms.

Calcarea carbonica (calcium carbonate)
> This remedy picture describes a woman who is obese and shows marked perspiration on her face and scalp. Her breasts are swollen and, although there is a free flow of milk, her baby cries and refuses to suckle. As a result, the mother commonly has tears silently trickling down her face.
> Using the 30c potency, give one dose only.

Lac caninum (dog's milk)
> This is a powerful remedy that may cause the milk to dry up completely. For this reason, use the 6c potency and give one dose only.

3. Loss of breast milk

The woman should be encouraged to drink plenty of fluid and reduce the amount of exercise that she is doing.

The following homoeopathic remedies can be used to help promote breast milk production. Select one by matching its picture with the clinical symptoms.

Using the 6c potency, give one dose, twice a day, for a maximum of twelve doses.

Agnus castus (chaste tree)

This remedy is the first choice of treatment. In the remedy picture, it describes a woman whose breast milk is drying up and she is particularly sad.

Lac defloratum (skimmed milk)

This remedy picture describes a woman who has a loss of breast milk with her breast size diminishing. She may also be experiencing throbbing headaches which are associated with a profuse flow of urine.

Pulsatilla (wind-flower)

This remedy picture describes a mother who is tearful and feels worse in hot, stuffy rooms. She prefers the fresh air and has her windows wide open.

4. Mastitis

This is caused by a blockage in a milk duct. It is treated by keeping the breast well supported, day and night, and by offering the affected breast first to her baby when the baby wants a feed.

The following homoeopathic remedies can be used to help alleviate the condition. Select the remedy whose picture most closely matches the clinical symptoms. Using the 6c potency, give one dose, twice a day for a maximum of twelve doses.

Belladonna (deadly nightshade)

This remedy picture describes a mother who has engorgement with an over-production of breast milk. Her breasts, or one of her breasts, are inflamed and tender to touch. She probably has a flushed face and may have a fever.

Bryonia (wild hops)

This remedy picture describes breast pains that are made worse by the slightest movement that is eased by rest.

This remedy can be used to follow on from *Belladonna* in helping to resolve any residual mastitis.

Hepar sulphuris (Hahnemann's calcium sulphide)

This remedy picture describes a breast that has a single area of abscess. The mother is unduly irritable and thirsty, craving sour fluids, especially vinegar. She also tends to sweat profusely and the sweat has an acutely offensive smell.

Phytolacca (poke root)

This remedy picture describes a breast with mastitis that is hard and lumpy. The mother has tender axillary lymph glands that drain the affected breast. Pressure on the nipple of the affected breast causes pain to be referred over the woman's entire body.

Silicea (pure flint)

This remedy picture describes a breast with mastitis where the nipple has become cracked. The mother feels totally exhausted. This remedy can be used to follow on from *Hepar sulphuris* in resolving any residual mastitis.

Use the same dosage schedule mentioned at the beginning of this section.

CHAPTER 10

INFANT DIFFICULTIES IN THE NEONATAL PERIOD

Remedies can be given to babies in granular, powder or liquid form. There is no therapeutic difference between these forms. The advantage of using homoeopathic remedies is that the baby need not be awoken, in order to give the medication, as the remedy can be put on the lips or exposed tongue.

One dose using granules is approximately 10 granules, and one drop of the liquid form equals one dose.

1. Post labour remedies

Arnica (leopard's bane)
>This remedy should be given in all cases of a difficult or prolonged labour, where there has been much moulding of the baby's head. Using the 30c potency, give a single dose.

Natrum sulphuricum (sodium sulphate)
>This remedy is to be used where the baby's head has been subjected to trauma, like a forceps delivery.
>Using the 30c potency, give a single dose.

2. Feeding difficulties

Accurate clinical diagnosis is essential so that the best course of therapy can be adopted. Homoeopathic remedies MUST be used only in a complementary role with conventional therapies.

Select the remedy by matching its picture with the clinical symptoms of the baby. Using the 30c potency, give one dose, daily, for a maximum of three doses.

Acid phosphoricum (phosphoric acid)
>This remedy picture describes a baby who is a slow feeder and consequently fails to thrive. The skin is pale and waxy; just not looking healthy. The baby has a tendency to lie in the cot with eyes wide open but not crying.

Aethusa cynapium (fool's parsley)
>This remedy picture describes a baby who vomits/regurgitates milk as soon as it has been swallowed. The baby remains hungry and, as a result, is clearly distressed.

Calcarea carbonica (calcium carbonate)
>This remedy picture describes the larger baby who also has a large head. Sweating is pronounced, particularly on their occiput. The baby is greedy but tends to vomit after a feed.

Natrum carbonicum (sodium carbonate)
>This remedy picture describes a baby who finds any form of milk disagreeable, leading to diarrhoea and regurgitation. Their abdomen becomes bloated and they pass a lot of flatus.

Silicea (pure flint)
>This remedy picture describes a small baby who has fine hair. The baby behaves contrarily by refusing the breast and yet, paradoxically, wanting it. The baby appears to be thirsty and accepts a bottle feed but, disappointingly, vomits it up after drinking from it.

3. Abdominal colic

Diagnosis is again important as colic can mask an acute abdomen, which requires urgent conventional treatment. Having been satisfied that there is no acute problem, then the following homoeopathic remedies can be used.

Select the remedy by matching its picture with the clinical symptoms. Using the 6c potency, give one dose as required.

Bryonia (wild hops)
>This remedy picture describes abdominal pains that are worsened by any pressure and only eased by absolute rest.

Carbo vegetabilis (vegetable charcoal)
>This remedy picture describes colicky pains occurring in a very windy baby, who has both flatulence and flatus.

Chamomilla (German chamomile)
>This remedy picture describes a baby whose pains make it very irritable and restless and it can only be pacified by being carried

around. Typically, one of their cheeks is red whilst the other is pale and cold. Their abdomen is distended with much flatus.

Colocynthis (bitter cucumber)
>This remedy picture describes a baby whose legs are drawn upwards whenever their colic occurs. Their colic pains are relieved by firm pressure.

Nux vomica (poison nut)
>This remedy picture describes a baby who develops colicky pains whenever they become over-tired. They have difficulty in defecating but the passage of a stool temporarily relieves their pain. An umbilical hernia is commonly present.

4. Septic spots

The following homoeopathic remedies can be used instead of antibiotics.

Select the remedy by matching its picture with the clinical symptoms. Using the 30c potency, give one dose, daily, for a maximum of three days.

Belladonna (deadly nightshade)
>This remedy picture describes skin that is red and showing the beginning of papules and is of particular use in the early stages of septic spot formation.

Hepar sulphuris (Hahnemann's calcium bisulphate)
>This remedy picture describes a later stage where pustules have actually formed.

Silicea (pure flint)
>This remedy picture describes a chronic situation. It is of use following the above two remedies in helping to resolve the infection, if progress has become static.

5. Sticky eyes

The following homoeopathic remedies can be used instead of antibiotic eye drops. They are given orally, using the 30c potency. Give one dose, daily, for a maximum of three days.

Argentum nitricum (silver nitrate)
> This remedy picture describes discharge from the baby's eyes that is often accompanied by oedema (swelling) of the conjunctiva.

Apis mellifica (honey bee)
> This remedy picture describes a picture where the actual eyelids of the baby become swollen. This remedy can be used after *Argentum nitricum* (silver nitrate).

6. Night crying

The diagnosis of night crying is either because the baby is in pain, needs their nappy changing or that they are bored. Provided that the first two have been adequately dealt with and the baby has been stimulated, but still cries, then the following homoeopathic remedies can be used.

Select the remedy by matching its picture with the clinical symptoms. Using the 30c potency, give one dose.

Chamomilla (German chamomile)
> This remedy picture describes a baby who is only quietened by being carried around.

Nux vomica (poison nut)
> This remedy picture describes a baby who wakes up in the early hours seemingly hungry and yet is not pacified by feeding. The baby's crying may improve by the passage of flatus or a stool.

Phosphorus
> This remedy picture describes a baby who takes short naps, throughout the day and night, but is unable to settle for a long sleep.

BIBLIOGRAPHY

Boericke W.   Materia Medica with repertory
                      Boericke and Tafel Philadelphia 1927

Boyd H. W.   Introduction to Homoeopathic Medicine
                      Beaconsfield 1981

Gemmell D.   Everyday Homoeopathy
                      Beaconsfield 1987

Kent J. T.   Repertory of the Homoeopathic
                      Materia Medica
                      Homoeopathic Book Service 1986

Lockie A. H.   The Family Guide to Homoeopathy
                      Penguin Books London 1989

Treacher S.   Practical Homoeopathy
                      Paragon 1997

Webb P. J.   The Family Encyclopedia of Homoeopathic
                      Remedies
                      Robinson 1997

USEFUL INFORMATION AND ADDRESSES

National Health Service GPs can refer patients to homoeopathic consultants in the following NHS Homoeopathic hospitals:

The Royal London Homoeopathic Hospital NHS Trust,
Great Ormond Street, **London** WC1N 3HR

Tel: 0171 837 8833

Glasgow Homoeopathic Hospital,
W. Glasgow Hospital University NHS Trust,
1053 Great Western Road, **Glasgow** G12 0XQ

Tel: 0141 211 1600

Bristol Homoeopathic Hospital,
United Bristol NHS Trust,
Cotham Road, Cotham, **Bristol** BS6 6JU

Tel: 0117 973 1231

Tunbridge Wells Homoeopathic Hospital,
Kent & Sussex Weald NHS Trust,
Church Road, **Tunbridge Wells**, Kent, TN1 1JU

Tel: 01892 542977

Department of Homoeopathic Medicine,
The Old Swan Health Centre,
St. Oswald's Street, Old Swan, **Liverpool** L13 2BY

Tel: 0151 228 6808

Most chemists and health-food shops stock a limited range of homoeopathic remedies. For the full range of remedies, however, one has to go to a specialised pharmacy or direct to the manufacturer. All products can be supplied by post.

Ainsworths Homoeopathic Pharmacy,
36 New Cavendish Street, London, W1M 7LH   Tel: 0171 935 5330
Buxton and Grant,
176 Whiteladies Road, Bristol BS8 2XU   Tel: 0117 9735025
Freeman's,
7 Eaglesham Road, Clarkston Glasgow, G76 7BU

Tel: 0141 644 1165

Galen Homoeopathics,
Lewell mill, West Stafford, Dorchester, Dorset DT2 8AN
Tel: 01305 263996
Goulds,
14 Crowndale Road, London, NW1 1TT
Tel: 0171 388 4752 or 0171 387 1888
Helios Homoeopathic Pharmacy,
97 Camden Road, Tunbridge Wells, Kent, TN1 2QR
Tel: 01892 537254 (Ansaphone)
and 01892 536393
Jolleys Pharmacy,
36 Witton Street, Northwich, Cheshire, CW9 5AH
Tel: 01606 331552
Nelsons Homoeopathic Pharmacies,
73 Duke Street, London, W1M 6BY
Tel: 0171 495 2404
Weleda (UK) Ltd.,
Heanor Road, Ilkeston, Derbyshire, DE7 8DR
Tel: 0800 626107

Phials, storage boxes, unmedicated tablets and other homoeopathic supplies can be obtained by post from:
The Homoeopathic Supply Co.,
4 Nelson Road, Sheringham, Norfolk, NR26 8BU
Tel: 01263 824683

Biochemic Tissue Salts and combination remedies can generally be obtained from homoeopathic pharmacies, health-food shops and from some chemists, or directly from:
Seven Seas Ltd.,
Hedon Road, Marfleet, Hull, HU9 5NJ
Tel: 01482 375234

Bach Flower Remedies are stocked by homoeopathic pharmacies and some health-food shops, or can be bought from:
Bach Flower Remedies Ltd.,
Broadheath House, 83 Parkside, Wimbledon, London, SW19 5LP
Tel: 0171 495 2404

TRAINING

The Faculty of Homoeopathy, which was incorporated by an Act of Parliament in 1950, promotes the academic and scientific development of homoeopathy and regulates the education, training and practice of homoeopathy by doctors, veterinary surgeons, podiatrists, dentists, nurses, midwives, pharmacists and all statutorily registered health care professionals.

Introductory courses are available for statutorily registered health care professionals (eg. nurses, midwives etc.) to gain a basic understanding of homoeopathy enabling them to give informed guidance to patients, and apply homoeopathy in a targeted way in their patient care. Courses involve interdisciplinary learning and specialist training for individual disciplines. Some intermediate training is also available. Courses are held at Bristol, Glasgow and London, and statutorily registered health care professionals are eligible to sit the PHCE (Primary Health Care Examination).

For further information, contact:

Administrator - Academic Unit,
Faculty of Homoeopathy
Royal London Homoeopathic Hospital
Great Ormond Street, London, WC1N 3HR

Tel: 0171 837 8833

Other publications by the

British Homoeopathic Association
27A Devonshire Street, London W1N 1RJ
Tel: 0171 935 2163
include:

Children's Toybox
  by Dr. A. Wynne-Simmons
Children's Types
  by Dr. D. Borland
Elements of Homoeopathy
  by Dr. D. M. Gibson
The Family Encyclopedia of Homoeopathic Remedies
  by Dr. Peter Webb (published by Robinson)
First Aid Homoeopathy in Accidents and Ailments
  by Dr. D. M. Gibson
Homoeopathic Treatment in the Nursery
  by Dr. H. Fergie-Woods
Homoeopathy for Mother and Infant
  by Dr D. Borland

A wide selection of books on homoeopathy is available by post from the Association.

An Information Pack, including lists of doctors and veterinary surgeons practising homoeopathy, will be sent on receipt of a stamped (60p) self-addressed A4 envelope. Membership of the BHA is open to anyone interested in homoeopathy. Members receive the magazine 'HOMOEOPATHY', six times a year, and have access to the Burford Library.

INDEX

Abdominal symptoms 20, 40
abruptia placenta 28
after-pains 33
aggravation 3
anaemia 10, 11
analgesics in labour 32
anxiety 3, 9, 11, 13, 22, 25, 28, 30, 31

Backache 29, 32
Braxton Hicks' contractions 30
breast feeding difficulties 36

Candida albicans 18
chloasma 27
circulatory problems 23
colic 20
colic (infant) 40, 41
constipation 10, 20
constitutional remedy 3, 5, 6, 9, 28, 35
cracked nipple 36, 38
cramps 23, 24
cravings 21
cystitis 18

Ectopic pregnancy 10, 11
emotional difficulties 30
episiotomy 31, 32

Fainting 24
fatigue 5, 12
feeding difficulties (babies) 39
first trimester 10

Haemorrhoids 22, 23
heartburn 12
hydramnios 28
hypotonic uterine activity 32

Incontinence 19
infant difficulties 39

Labour 32, 35

Malpresentation 31
mastitis 37, 38
milk production
   (increased and decreased) 36, 37
miscarriage 12, 13, 14
morning sickness 12, 14, 15, 16

Neonatal period 39
night crying 42

Palpitations 25
phlebitis 25
piles (see haemorrhoids)
placenta praevia 28
post partum blues 32
post partum haemorrhage 34
potency 2
pre-eclampsia 28

Remedy pictures 3, 4, 5
retained placenta 34

Second trimester 17
septic spots 41
skin changes 27
sore nipples 36
sticky eyes 41
succussion 1

Third trimester 29
thrush, recurrent 18

Urogenital tract 17

Vaginal discharge 17, 18
varicose veins 23, 26, 27
vomiting (see morning
   sickness)
vulval damage 32